A REASONABLE REASON TO WAIT

*A Practical Guide for
Those Who Have Not Been
Sexually Involved and
Healing for Those Who Have*

BY
JACOB ARANZA
WITH
THERESA LAMSON

Copyright © Jacob Aranza, 1984
Printed in the United States of America
ISBN Number 0-910311-21-8

All rights reserved. No part of this book may be reproduced without permission from the publisher, except by a reviewer who may quote brief passages in a review; nor may any part of this book be reproduced, stored in a retrieval system or copied by mechanical, photocopying, recording or other means, without permission from the publisher.

The author expresses special thanks to Fred and Debbie Davis for their help with the manuscript.

To my lovely wife Michelle

My reason to wait

TABLE OF CONTENTS

INTRODUCTION

During the time we spent writing this book, many inquired as to its subject matter. When either of us mentioned its content, people often cringed. Some adults seem to think there aren't any moral problems in our society! But others remember the free love "flower children" from nearly two decades ago, who abruptly changed the moral views of the American public.

Those flower children have grown up, cut their hair, and now have families of their own. Their children now have to grow up in an amoral society; one without morals. No longer is there a moral standard for young people to look up to. The majority of teenagers are being forced to rise up and be some type of a standard, or have no morals at all!

Becoming amoral has gradually taken hold of our society over the past 20 years. While many sneer at the Moral Majority, the fact remains that most Americans (and Europeans for that matter) have been brainwashed into sub-standard morals or no morals at all. Television is now the new sex teaser of the western world. It promises to always go as far sexually as possible to keep us waiting for the next episode which will be seen (they tell us) at the same time on the same channel!

While thumbing through two recent copies of *T.V. Guide* magazine, I wondered if they were guides to television or guides to immorality. Who gets the best ratings? The network that can deliver a program with the best, the latest, or the hottest new sex symbol, will get the most viewers. America will cling to the program that helps them fantasize and escape from reality.

Television has delivered to us every scheme imaginable, pushing ethical limits as far as possible, with their skimpy bikinis and cleavage-showing dresses! They will deliver to us anything they can, short of full nudity and full sex. Those honors are left to the cable channels and can be bought for a small price! Along with other media, television is simply a reflection of the mental and physical appetites of the majority of Americans.

Is it any wonder that eight out of 10 people have lost their virginity by the age of 20? "Love" has been reduced to a simple physical act. Few young people understand the love that makes a lifetime marriage, because they don't see enough of it around them!

We, like the Roman and Greek civilizations, of

history, have finally elevated sex to a god-status. With America and Europe leading the way, the world has not only taken a moral landslide, but has shaken our individual basic convictions to the point of collapse! We have been smitten by such great moral decay, that our world has become evil as it was in the days of Noah (Luke 17:26).

It is our desire, therefore, in writing this book, that your own morality would be challenged and self-examined. The quotes, statistics and personal confessions that you will read in the pages to follow, are food for your thoughts. May Christ reveal the true intents of your heart as only He can!

FOR YOUR INFORMATION

★ 60% of the general public feel sex before marriage is okay.

★ 300,000 teenage abortions occur yearly.

★ 600,000 babies are born out of wedlock in America yearly.

★ 20 million people currently have the incurable herpes disease.

★ One out of four homes is predicted to have incest within it's walls.

★ 1,000 people have died from the fatal disease AIDS.

★ If current rape trends continue, one out of three twelve-year-old American girls will have been the victims of rape.

1

SEXLESS

Many of today's parents have liberal minds that don't think anything of buying concert tickets for their teenagers to go to see "The Police" or "Boy George." Of course, it's no wonder. A lot of these parents were taking acid in the 60s!

Popular music shows us what's really going on with our youth today. And I am really amazed at what I see! The music idols of today seem to be competing for the "who's the strangest" contest. We have entered into a trend of adrogyny — that is, having both male and female characteristics. I was overwhelmed to see a local costume event with half the guys dressed as Boy George! The most interesting thing about him is that he is not gay. Though he jokes about being a "drag queen," he swears it's all in fun. He claims to be quite masculine.[1]

We also have the likes of Michael Jackson, who looks like Dianna Ross in drag. He lives with his parents who insist he isn't gay either. And Annie Lennox, of the Eurythmics, says she dresses like a man as a joke!

Although people still find transsexuals a little hard to accept, we have become used to people playing a game with sex roles. We see films like Tootsie, Yentl, and Victor/Victoria which promote the fun and benefits of this game. Our clothing industry has women dressed in men's suits: with baggy pleated pants, and boxy double-breasted jackets.

You know we're really locking into this trend when Calvin Klein is expected to gross $70 million by the end of 1984 on a line of men's underwear for women. His string bikini for women looks like a jockey strap and the boxer shorts actually have a fly![2]

But it's not the rock stars, clothing designers, and hairdressers who are creating this change. It is a change in the way we're thinking, and the above industries are just trying to cooperate with the public!

One of the greatest thrills in this life is the thrill of anticipation. That's one reason why the "thriller" movies make it so big on the silver screen. They play on the fun of anticipation and people love it.

It's like the child who is always trying to grow up. His great joy is in doing something new to show how big he is and he'll lie awake at night in anticipation. But we have deeply abused this emotional activity and corrupted it.

We have turned our culture into one where you can get whatever you want, when you want it. We don't care how we affect others by our "wantsies"; we just take what we want and have a good time with it.

This attitude has spilled over into sexual pleasure. Sex once was something a young person had to look forward to. Now, it's no big thrill because everybody does it! It's just another activity to do, whenever you want to do it!

Sex has become so much a part of a young person's life, that our youth have had to look for something else that could be a new, exciting experience. For many young people, sex, like pot, is too trendy and they want something different. This has brought us punk rock, with it's violent slam-dancing and it's pins and needles. But, the less physical teens are clinging to the newer sexless idols. Many of our young people use these figures to escape the sexual pressure of their peers. Boy George is not sexually exciting! (Sorry, George!) But there is a sick sexuality about him, and our teenagers are simply trading one form of evil for another!

In understanding this, it is clear to see why I am asked over and over again, "How do I know if I'm in love?" How can teenagers understand true love when their idols are both male and female? How can they be sure if they're in love when the most intimate part of a marriage relationship is just another habit like brushing your teeth?

"Wherefore, God also gave them up to un-

*cleanness through the lusts of their own
hearts, to dishonor their own bodies between
themselves"* (Romans 1:24).

1 *People Magazine:* Apr. 23, 1984

2 *People Magazine:* Apr. 23, 1984

2

RATED X

Americans are just beginning to understand how strong an influence the media has on us. So often I've heard the Christian say, "Oh, there was a lot of cussing in the movie, but I just ignored it." This person doesn't realize how sharp the mind is. It doesn't miss a trick!

The sensitive Christian who sees a movie with bad language in it, will leave the theatre feeling hassled, or at least a little aggravated! Not that we can't handle bad language, but it works against our spiritual nature.

So often I'll be discouraged to hear young Christains talking about movies in the following way: "Yeah . . . I went to see 'An Officer and a Gentleman'." A friend replies, "Wasn't that rated R?" "Well", he says, "it just had some bad language

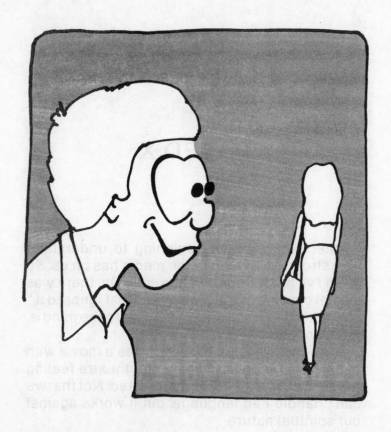

and a few sex scenes. But the rest of it was great."

Another time a husband and wife told me about the time they went to see an R-rated movie. "We went to see '48 Hours'. We thought it was rated R because it was a police story and we figured it was violent." Little did they know that every other word would be sexually suggestive and vulgar! I don't know why we sat through the whole thing! By the time we left we both were so drained from trying to block out all the filth! It really cured us from going to see R-rated films!"

I wish it were just the R-rated films we had to worry about, that would make life simple. But the ones now rated PG are the type of films that were rated R, when I was growing up! You never know, when you go to see a PG film, if it's rated PG because of one violent scene, or because it's sex from start to end!

The only way I go to movies anymore is if I see what the reviews say, or hear someone talk about it. I've even asked an unsaved person if they've seen one so I could find out what it is about! We have to learn to keep ourselves away from bad influences! And, in this day and age, we have to work harder at it! What we keep feeding our minds is what we will come to accept as normal.

One young man I know told me, "I just went to see 'Class' and, man was it great." When I asked him what it was about he said, "Oh, it's about a guy who has an affair with his friend's mother." "Sounds real wholesome," I sarcastically said.

Now, I'm not about to tell you to stop going to the movies; though I will say that those who don't

go to them are doing themselves a great service!
But I will say to you, BEWARE! You won't be able
to control your sexuality if you go to see movies
that are full of flesh and sex. Be honest and admit
that a great majority of them are that way!

Find out what a movie is about before you consider going to see it. People talk about movies so
often, that it isn't hard to find out about them. We
even have television shows that review movies.
Don't go to see something that you know is going
to have a lot of sex, or a sexual theme. I mean,
come on, the title "First Turn On" gives you fair
enough warning!

Take a stand against movies that are rated R.
You won't be missing out on anything but you will
receive God's blessing for choosing what is right.
And be extra cautious, because what is now rated
PG was once rated R. And what is now rated R
should be rated X!

3

MISUNDERSTOOD BIBLE SEX WORDS

Many people, especially those just entering adulthood, find it difficult to believe that there are words in the Bible that deal with every facet of a relationship between two members of the opposite sex. Many young people have told me that they didn't even know that sex before marriage was condemned by the Bible!

I was recently getting my hair cut and ended up in a conversation with a young lady in her late teens who expressed this viewpoint to me. She was religious and attended weekly church services. Finally she blurted out, "Is sex before marriage REALLY a sin?"

Many find Bible words relating to sex just to be other spiritual words they don't understand. This is why the Bible says, "Study to show thyself ap-

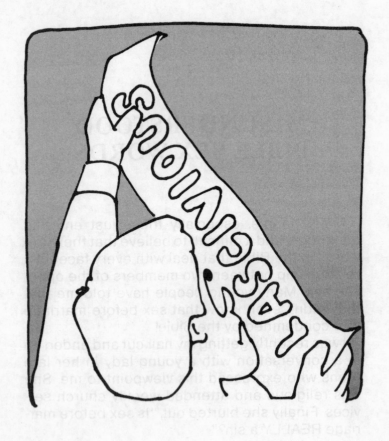

proved . . ." (2 Tim. 2:15).

Many times we must study words to understand their meaning and the following are just such words.

LASCIVIOUSNESS

This word is sometimes translated "sexuality" in the sense to "choose to stir yourself up sexually," outside of God's limits. For the Christian this is usually the result of a lack of discipline.

Lasciviousness can be accomplished a number of ways. One method is through the means of pornography. The sight of someone naked stimulates (or turns on) a person sexually and causes them to try and satisfy this sexual urge. This same sexual arousal can come through suggestive movies or pornographic books.

But the main way that many are involved in lasciviousness is through masturbation. In a recent survey of over 100,000 women, well over 80% said they masturbated, and most of them did it frequently.[1] In these findings, 54% of the women started masturbating by the age of 15 and 32% between the ages of 10 to 15! In another survey, 86% of the males under 24 years of age claimed to masturbate.[2] The statistics may seem shocking, but all recent surveys prove these figures to be true.

In Galatians 5:17 we find lasciviousness mentioned, and in verse 21 Paul warns that those who are involved in it will not inherit the Kingdom of God! Clearly this is VERY important to God!

EVIL CONCUPISCENCE

This term is used three times in the Bible. Twice it is used regarding sexual passion. Interpreted "evil desire" or "lustful passion," it means to have an abnormal or uncontrollable sexual appetite. This relates to a constant habit; whether through thoughts, actions, or speech. But, whatever the form, people involved in evil concupiscence are controlled by their sex drives.

One example of this type of problem is the person who has a "dirty mind." With this habit of the mind the person constantly thinks about everything in sexual terms. This type of person makes others feel uncomfortable and can make you feel like you're being examined or X-rayed!

In 1 Thessalonians 4:5 Paul speaks to the church and forbids them to be involved in concupiscence. In Col. 3:5,6 he tells the church that this sin results in the wrath of God being placed on the children of disobedience. This little sin of pleasure will receive a harse judgement!

DEFRAUD

The word "defraud" is used to describe someone who has been taken advantage of. In 1 Thessalonians 4:6 we are warned against this and that it, too, is worthy of the wrath of God!

The next scripture in this passage says, "... for God has not called us to impurity, but to purity...". Defrauding, or taking advantage of someone sex-

ually, happens when we sexually arouse someone with our actions or how we dress ourselves.

The person who wears jeans so tight you can
read the date on the dime in the back pocket is, in
fact, defrauding others! So is the female who
wears blouses that draw attention to her breasts.
And the list goes on and on... bikinis... short-cut
shorts ... etc. These are all forms of sexually defrauding people! The sad thing about it is that a lot
of Christians that dress this way aren't even a-
ware of what they're doing to other people. And
some don't even care! But many don't realize that
they're causing people to lust after them.

Another way people sexually defraud one another is by necking, or making out. Too often the
story goes that "necking" is okay when you're
dating. After all, they say, they've got it "under
control." But being "under control" is not the
problem.

The problem is that any sexual arousal, outside
of the marriage relationship, is defrauding and an
abomination to God. This is a hard truth for the
young and in-love to swallow! But it is the Word of
God and, rest assured, that what He says is harm-
ful for you, He will give you the strength to over-
come.

For instance, one couple told me that they each,
individually, were full of sexual sin before knowing the Lord. When they came to know the Lord
and started dating each other, they didn't even
hold hands until a short time before their marriage, because they knew how easy it would be to
get carried away. They didn't want to take the
chance of ruining the great relationship God had

given them! And they'll be the first to tell you that it's not always easy!

But they'll also tell you that, because they didn't want to sin, God has made the sexual part of their marriage far more enjoyable than anything they had experienced in the past, before knowing Christ.

Obedience to God's word ALWAYS brings rewards and happiness! He is a rewarder of those who diligently seek Him (Hebrews 11:6).

FORNICATION

Most of the time when fornication is used in the Bible it refers to sex between two unmarried people. But it is also used to talk about a sexually unfaithful husband or wife, more commonly called adultery or extra-marital sex.

The scripture warns many times that we are to stay away from fornication and not be involved in sexual sin. In 1 Thessalonians, again we are warned that God will be the avenger or judge, for all who are involved in it.

One thing that each of these words has in common is that they begin in the mind.

Someone once said, "If you plant a thought, you will reap an action. If you plant an action, you will reap a habit. If you plant a habit, you will reap a destiny for that habit; life or death, heaven or hell."

In this way the mind is like the stomach. Whatever you feed it most is what it will have the greatest appetite for. What are you feeding your mind?

Television? Movies? Pop or rock music? Seventy-five percent of all of those are tied to sex! No wonder our thoughts so often are impure!

When we understand the ways of the world, along with understanding the Bible words we just discussed, we realize that the only way we can keep ourselves from these sexual problems is to clean up our acts! We have to make a mental decision to fill our minds with clean thoughts. That's why we're told, in Philippians 4, to fill our minds with good, healthy, honest, and pure thoughts.

Cleaning up our minds is not an easy task. A lot of us are used to thinking one way. And, many of us have people around us hassling us with filth. But if the Bible says it can be done ... IT CAN BE DONE ... One step at a time! Make that first step today.

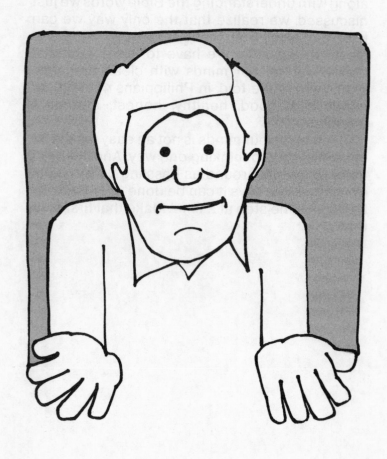

4

YOU'VE BEEN ROBBED!

An excuse that is often used to justify premarital sex is that the couple is planning to get married. For the girl, especially, this eases the guilt. For a guy, it's the greatest line invented since the telephone!

Recent statistics show as many as eight out of 10 couples are sexually involved with one another before their wedding night. Could this be one of the main reasons behind the high divorce rate?

It is well documented that couples who have been involved with each other before marriage trust each other less than couples who waited for marriage.

Why do you think this is? The reason is simple. If my marriage partner jumped the fence to be involved with me, what will keep him or her from jumping the fence again with someone else?

God's plan is to bless sex through the marriage relationship. And those who wait until their wedding night will receive a special blessing from God. This may seem crazy to our natural minds. What difference does this make when you *know* you're getting married anyway? Let's see.

It reminds me of Christmas.

When I was growing up I remember cheating and opening my presents when no one was around. Then I'd close them up and wait until Christmas. I'll never forget trying to look surprised on Christmas day when I opened them! And I'd always feel guilty. I'd spoiled my own fun.

Actually, I'd been robbed! I'd been robbed of the true joy that was intended for me by my parents. I had broken the rules.

In the same way our Heavenly Father has a rule for the wedding day. The special present is your wife or husband. And, if you wait until your wedding day, the joy you have will be a great blessing. If you don't wait, your wedding night will be spoiled and you will have been robbed!

There is a great difference between Christmas and your wedding! Christmas gives you temporary joy. Your wedding gives you a marriage that changes the rest of your life. I can think of so many times I've counseled couples whose marriages were either totally destroyed or had problems that were tied to the fact that they had premarital sex.

One such couple was Chuck and Terry. They were a very attractive couple and, when I first met them, they were living together. I remember when they first decided to get married. She was so happy and they were so in love.

After they were married everything seemed to be going great until he began to work long hours. Soon, she found a boyfriend. What happened to their relationship is very common. They released a monster in their relationship before they were ever married. It was the monster of mistrust and unfaithfulness. They were unfaithful to God before marriage. This had opened the door to be unfaithful to one another.

Another result from premarital sex is the case of Bob and Marion. They had sex before marriage and she walked down the aisle about three months pregnant. Their marriage has never been right. She has always resented Bob and has felt guilty about this sin. She won't forgive him and she won't forgive herself. They now have two children.

Bob and Marion never do things together. They always seem to be doing their own thing. It's hard to remember that, when they were first dating, they were like best friends and never were seen apart!

Still another result was a girl named Laura. The first time I ever spoke at her church I saw her standing out in the crowd. She was one of those beautiful girls who looked like she just stepped out of a fashion magazine. Her bright blue eyes and warm smile always drew attention.

Laura and Rob had been going steady for about three years and they soon would be married. Just before the wedding date everyone began noticing her gaining weight. This was not at all like the petite Laura everyone knew. The wedding day came and went. Seven months later she had a baby.

Nearly a year later someone told me they had seen Laura out shopping. She had cut off her long beautiful hair and weighed about 175 pounds. Not long after that she was treated for an alcohol problem.

I heard a man tell a story recently about a woman in his church. Everytime an altar call was made for people who needed prayer she would step forward weeping. This would occur continually.

The pastor finally asked, "Why do you come up week after week?"

The woman answered with her head down, "Twenty years ago my husband and I were involved sexually before we were married and I've never been able to forgive myself."

So often it is the women who suffer with guilt. And, like Laura, often they eat a lot of guilt.

These once beautiful girls become fat and sloppy. Their self-identity is ruined.

That's a high price to pay for one night of pleasure!

Because guys aren't as emotional as girls are, they often put the pressure on their girlfriends for sex. This is unfair to the girls who so badly want the acceptance of their boyfriends.

Almost every girl would wait until marriage to have sex if it weren't for the pressure of their boyfriends.

But I'm not placing all the blame on the guys. It works both ways.

If you girls don't want sexually pushy boyfriends

then you'd better keep your hands off their thighs and your kisses off their necks! And you can check your wardrobe, too.

If you two are in-love, he will love you for who you are on the inside, not for how exciting you look on the outside!

On the other hand, you guys have to reassure your girlfriends that you love them for who they are so they don't feel like they have to be impressing you all the time.

"But what if we don't get along sexually? Wouldn't it be better to make sure before we decided if we are 'right' for each other?"

I've had those questions asked, too. And the answer is quite simple. The bodies of men and women are made to join together. There is no way that they couldn't be "right" for each other.

The question I'm really being asked is what if my partner likes sex one way and I like it another way?

Sex, like any other part of marriage, is something you grow into. It's a learning experience for both people, a giving and taking. When you really love your husband/wife, you want to do what pleases them and vice-versa. You learn to tell each other what you do and don't like. It's not like the passion they show on T.V. where it looks like every couple is in ecstasy!

It's much better than that. You're getting to know each other intimately and can have a lot of fun in the process!

There are even some good Christian books out that teach you about how God made our bodies.

On several occasions I have given a copy to

newlyweds and advised them to read it together. In each case I was thanked and told how much it helped them.

One couple took it on their honeymoon and sent me a thank-you card. This type of book can really help take the fear out of this new experience in your relationship.

I remember one guy's excuse for premarital sex: "Would you buy a pair of shoes without trying them on first?"

I wonder how that made his girlfriend feel?

The "Dear Abby" section of our local newspaper answered one such question.

A girl wrote in and said, "Dear Abby, My boyfriend wants me to have sex with him but I told him I wanted to wait until I was married first. He said, 'How would I ever know I didn't like sex before marriage if I never tried it'?"

Dear Abby responded, "Tell him to try gargling cement. How does he know he won't like it if he's never tried it?!"

If you are going to get married, below are some questions you need to ask yourself and the person you're going to marry.

1. *Do you want to risk the chance of allowing guilt to ruin your identities, or lose your respect for each other?*

2. *Do you want to take the risk of missing out on God's blessing*

on your marriage?

3. *Since you're getting married anyway, can't you care enough about your relationship to wait and make your wedding day a very special day in your lives to remember?*

4. *Should you take the risk of not being able to trust each other?*

After you've asked yourself these questions, think them through and talk about them. If you're honest with each other, you will decide to wait.

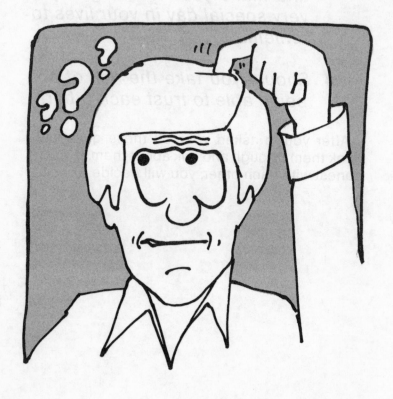

5

WHAT ABOUT ME?

Once we've passed that strange stage called puberty, we're suddenly young adults who *physically* can start families.

Guys are no longer grossed-out at the thought of kissing a girl; and girls are shocked to find out that one wink of the eye can draw her more than ordinary attention from a young man!

It's both an age full of fun and full of danger.

Communications is one key factor in making teenage years happy ones. If a teenager has an adult they can talk to, a lot of problems can be spared them.

But the adults (hopefully the parents) have to be good listeners.

Young people have minds of their own and are trying to shape their morals and goals. If they can trust an adult or parent enough to tell them their ideas, they'll respect and trust their advice.

They must be allowed to think through their ideas and then come to the right conclusions.

I've seen it work this way time and time again. The teenager has kept his or her identity while receiving direction through the parents' experience.

But what if you're a teenager and you don't have the parent or adult who wants to hear your point of view?

Unfortunately, you're going to have to grow up much faster than your friends!

If you think differently than your parents, that's okay. But, as long as you're in their house, you must abide by their rules.

Some teenagers think that if they leave home early, then they can live life their own way. It's only then that they find out how hard it is to support themselves and how cruel the real world can be!

Enjoy the freedom your parents provide you with! Maybe abiding by their rules seems hard, but it's no comparison to what you'll have to face the rest of your life once you leave their home!

We have to discuss the three vital areas of need that must be met in every young person's life.

If these needs aren't met at home, the boy or girl will search somewhere else to fill them and they'll find them in the opposite sex.

ACCEPTANCE

Every young person must feel that they are valuable and accepted by their family and their friends. Acceptance is one of the greatest motivations that exists.

It is very important that parents openly show acceptance to their children.

Teenagers don't take it lightly when they're kidded for having acne, big feet, or a changing voice. Adults will often talk like they're 'objects' instead of human beings.

The parents don't mean any harm and very often are just speaking out of the awe of watching their child become an adult! But this type of kidding can be very damaging to the teenager.

The young person who is secure in his acceptance at home isn't dependent on the acceptance of his friends at school or elsewhere.

APPROVAL

Approval is one of the greatest slave drivers of all time. It will take a person and never let him go until he feels as though he is finally a success in the eyes of others.

I remember talking to a college basketball coach. He told me a story about one of his players.

When this guy was in high school he had all the qualities that make a pro: the height, speed and jumping ability.

But he was not playing up to his potential because his family never came to see him play. He never received encouragement from them. When they finally went to see him play, in his senior year, he became the top scorer and rebounder!

The approval of his family gave him the confidence he needed to be his best.

I'm not saying here that your parents must approve of your sin. But, just as Jesus loved the sinner and hated the sin, teenagers need to be approved, encouraged and loved as individuals.

AFFECTION

Affection is probably the most important of the three A's I am talking about.

I remember the day my dad and I were walking through downtown Houston. He reached out to hold my hand as we crossed the busy central business area. But I didn't want to hold his hand. Soon, I didn't want my mom kissing me anymore.

What was wrong? I was getting affection somewhere else. I was becoming more interested in the affection of the opposite sex.

Teenagers, especially, have an appetite for affection. This need must be fed. When young people stop wanting affection at home, they're probably getting it somewhere else. Their fathers are the most important male figures during these years. They need to be hugged and held, especially in the early teens.

Boys need affection as well but have a great need for approval. They tend to be more accomplishment-oriented and must know when they have done well.

Many fathers, who have insecurity problems themselves, find it difficult to show approval to their sons. Fathers should never let their past determine their son's future!

I can recall many counseling sessions where I've wondered just how many of these qualities were instilled in the teenagers.

One time there was a young girl who came to one of my crusades. She had taken all of her rock records and broken them, symbolizing a new start and change in her life.

A year later her parents had asked me to counsel her. I hardly recognized her with her faded jeans and her punk haircut. As I shook hands with her mom and dad, she sat down looking like she was awaiting torture! Her wild rebellious look seemed alien to the beautiful girl I once knew.

Her parents began to tell me how their model daughter had begun to destroy her life. They talked of the conflicts she was having with the other girls at school. The story climaxed by telling of the punk rock boyfriend that she had run away with to spend the night.

"Where have we gone wrong?," the mother asked. "We've tried to do what was right and fair," the calm, but stern father added.

Her parents soon left the room so I could speak to the girl in private.

As soon as the door closed I looked directly into the face of a young, bewildered girl, torn between loyalties to her family and her newly found boyfriend.

I calmly asked, "What's going on?"

"Well my parents and I had a fight over my music and punk clothes. So I ran away to my boyfriend's house and we spent the night together."

It didn't sound like either party was a very good listener!

There are no pat answers to such problems and how they've developed. Each situation is different and must be handled on an individual basis.

But I will say that communication and the three A's (affection, approval, and acceptance), when provided at home, are the greatest prescriptions in keeping a teenager from giving in to peer pressure.

What about me? I need love and affection, acceptance, approval and someone to talk to!

6

LOOKING FOR LOVE

How did you fall in love?

Where did you meet your boyfriend or girl-friend?

How do you spend your time together?

These are some very important questions you need to ask yourself.

"I first saw him at a party and thought he was cute," is a common reply; or, "When I saw her in class I thought she was such a fox!"

What deep qualities!

These are the thoughts of a generation that thinks, "What you see is what you get."

But, the truth is, you can have a person with a beautiful body on the outside, but is a lying, cheating, hateful person on the inside.

We've got a society that *loves* what it looks at!

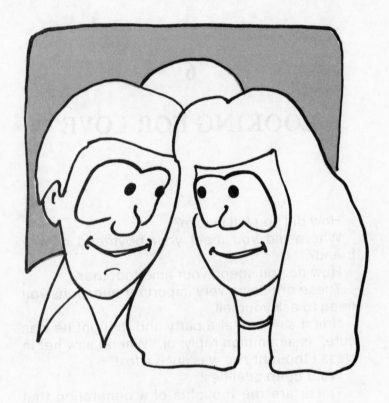

We really worship the body.

As a result we get people like John.

He wants to marry a girl with blond hair and blue eyes. But what about that red-head who would give her life for him?

Forget it!

It is even worse than that.

If he has acne, or zits, hang it up! Or if she doesn't wear Espirit, she's not for me!

We love people because of who they are on the outside.

If you love someone because of their great figure, what happens to that love when their figure changes?

If you love that guy with the great build, what happens to that love when his great build turns into a great bulge in his belly?

Our culture is ruled by physical attraction. We seem to think physical attraction lasts forever. At least, that's what the T.V. soaps make us think!

Since our world judges everything by how it looks on the outside, we don't expect people to look beyond that. This is a "plastic love," it's not real; it won't stand the test of time.

So many young girls are looking for a real love but all they get is this cheap plastic stuff!

I recently heard a girl say, "All guys give you is junk sex and it's not much better than junk food!"

These girls end up confused and hurt because they were fooled into thinking the experience was a lasting love.

But the real, lasting love wants what's best for the other person. It doesn't think of itself.

I remember the time I met Susan.

She went to a private school where she was a popular cheerleader. I had helped a friend of her's who was sexually involved, so she asked me to come talk with her.

I sat down in her living room and looked down at the large family Bible on her parents' coffee table. After talking a few minutes about school, I asked her what she really wanted to talk to me about.

She looked down and answered, "Well I guess you know I've been kinda involved with my boyfriend."

"Yes," I answered.

She started crying.

When I finally looked up at me, she said, "We're really in love, you know. We really do love each other."

Then, as we continued to talk, Susan admitted that she felt ashamed before God. She knew it really wasn't right.

I explained to her that God would forgive her and change her life if she would open up her heart to Him and ask his forgiveness. She decided to turn to Jesus that very day and I prayed with her. Susan promised to meet me at church the following Tuesday.

That Tuesday night I waited outside of the church for her. I could hardly wait to see how she was doing in her new committment to Christ. When I realized she wasn't coming, I went in and called her house. Sure enough, she answered the phone and I asked her why she wasn't at church.

My boyfriend is here and he says that what you told me is wrong. We love each other, so it's okay for us to be involved," she said.

Next I heard her boyfriend's voice. "This is Allen. Are you the guy who told Susan I didn't love her?"

"Yes," I answered. "If you really loved her, you wouldn't be taking advantage of her."

After a moment of silence, he roughly said, "But I DO love her and that's why it's alright."

I asked him if he had ever been involved sexually with anyone else before Susan.

"That's none of your business!" he yelled.

I continued, "Did you love her, too?"

The next voice I heard was Susan's telling me that she didn't care to see me or talk to me again and that I had confused her.

Allen didn't want Susan to know that she was just another girl with whom he was temporarily "in love."

A year and a half later our youth group was out witnessing on a main drag that was a hangout for teenagers. We saw a car wreck and I went over to it. The wreck wasn't serious and I saw a teenage girl at the wheel, crying.

When I got a closer look, I was surprised.

"Susan, what are you doing?," I said.

She realized it was me and said, "Allen and I started going together again and I was looking for him. You haven't seen him, have you?"

"No," I told her, "I'm sorry, but I haven't."

When I walked away from that car I thought about how Susan was still chasing after someone who would give her attention and spend time with her. Like many other girls today, she was looking for love. But all she got was sex.

Allen, like many other young men, was willing to

give her just enough time and attention to get sex. I was sad to think of the pretty girl who was being fooled with "plastic love."

Thousands upon thousands of young girls believe this is real love!

I know it seems like I place all the blame on the guys. But, out of the countless teenagers I counsel, it's the girl who most often is being fooled and used.

Every once in awhile I come across a guy who is really serious about the girl. And sex, for this couple, is just a lack of self-control. If they understood true love, they wouldn't put themselves in places where they'd be tempted to have sex!

Another typical example is that of a girl named Carol.

She was both physically and mentally mature at a young age. Carol's dad was one of the finest Christian men I had ever known. Her parents gave her everything possible to see that her life was comfortable.

When we were first introduced, I went aside with Carol to get to talk with her in private. Most of our conversation concerned a guy by the name of Dan. With the way she talked about him, he seemed to be a south Texas blend of Tom Selleck, Robert Redford and the Incredible Hulk!

"I really do love him," she said.

I had to admit it was hard to believe!

"I know you've heard other girls say it before, but this really is different," she continued. "Just because I'm 14 doesn't mean I don't know what love is." After her long explanation of how wonderful and kind Dan was, I asked if she and Dan were involved physically.

In a soft voice she answered, "Yes, but Dan would never tell anyone."

I looked into her eyes and said, "Carol, if he didn't he'll be the first guy I ever met who never told anyone."

She defended her 16 year old king and angrily said, "You'll see; he's not like all the others!"

The next day, after I spoke at the local high school, Carol walked toward me with someone walking slowly behind her.

With a smile she said, "Jacob, I want you to meet Dan."

"Hi, Dan," I said, reaching out to shake his hand, while trying to give a warm smile.

Looking at Carol, and then back at me, he said, "Could I talk with you alone?"

Carol stood still as we began to walk away from the school.

"Carol says that you told her I tell other guys what we do in private," he said nervously.

"Well, do you?" I asked. "Well . . . only my closest friends," he replied.

I thought to myself, "If Carol could only hear him now!"

I began to think of all the other Carols who had believed the same old story! It's just a game, full of lies. How long would it be until these girls began to see this "plastic love" for what it really is? The sex they thought was "terms of endearment" was only "germs of endearment!"

So many young girls are so desperately looking for love that they won't believe the truth.

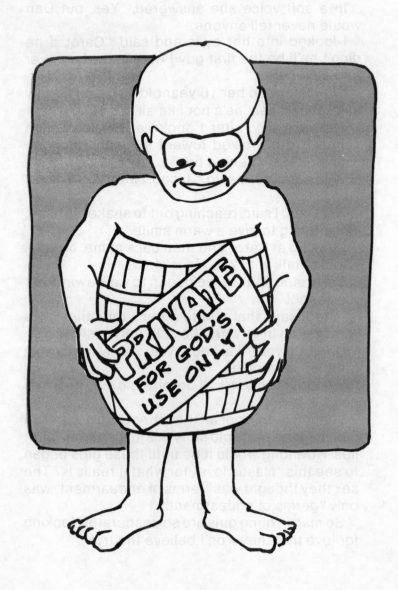

7

ALIVE AND WELL

Have you ever felt that you were in love with someone and your parents told you it was "puppy love?"

Why is it when a teenager feels this is love that the adult thinks they're too young for it to be real?

All during the teenage years, your ideas, likes, and dislikes are changing.

The 13 year old who wouldn't touch vegetables can easily become a vegetarian by his or her 18th birthday! That's because the way you think is changing at a fast speed.

Your senses have become super-active and will be for some time. You'll never again have the same energy you have as a teenager! Nothing matches it and no one knows it better than your parents! You're so "alive" right now that sometimes you get mad at older people because they seem to be moving slowly. It's not that they're doing things so slowly, but it's that you're running at top speed!

But the most noticeable thing happening is that you're becoming a young man or woman. When you start to have affectionate feelings for someone of the opposite sex it is easy to think it is love. After all, you've never felt quite that way about someone before.

So parents call it "puppy love" because it's a new experience for you. They *expect* your feelings to change, and for good reasons. They know that the kind of love that leads to marriage thinks more about the other person's needs than your own. And young people usually haven't developed this kind of love. Love, in marriage, is something you constantly work at. You, as a young adult, are not expected to "work" at your relationships in this way.

It's alright to have someone special in your life. I really have nothing against dating. But it's not wise to spend a lot of time alone with someone of the opposite sex. It's too easy to get physical and too hard to control these feelings once they get aroused.

The world is telling you "Hey, sex is fun!"

They make it look like a sport! We even read bumper stickers about it! They think, "Of course you're not going to marry THAT person, you're just out having some fun with them."

What the world doesn't tell you is that you're ruining your lives!

Maybe you have thought about getting pregnant so you go on birth control pills. But you haven't thought about feeling guilty or ruining things for your future marriage. Just think what it would be like to be married to someone who had a serious sexual relationship with someone else!

The world doesn't care about what the Bible says, but what it says *is true*.

For instance, the Bible says that when two people are joined together they become "one flesh." Something spiritual takes place when two people have sex, even though we don't completely understand it. What we *do* understand is that this union is blessed by God in marriage. When it's non-Christian, or outside of marriage, it becomes like a curse!

It's like the dating couple who are involved sexually and seem to always be breaking up and getting back together again, over and over and over! They're unhappy together and unhappy apart!

So often I've talked to girls who don't know why they can't seem to break up with the guys even though they're unhappy with them. I truly believe this has to do with their sexual union. Then, when they finally do break up, it's full of heartache. They have to tear apart that union, as unholy as it is!

Then what are we supposed to do when we really like and care for someone? Are we supposed to wait until we grow into the type of love for marriage?

If you feel strongly about someone of the opposite sex, then spend most of your time with them among other Christians.

The Bible doesn't even have the word "dating"

in it. Our concept of dating is a product of modern America! But the Bible does talk about "fellowship" which is being with other Christians.

It means hanging around other Christians who feel the same way about the Lord. The best way to get to know someone of the opposite sex is in fellowship. Do things as a group. Don't single yourself out with your boyfriend or girlfriend. You can't afford the luxury of temptation! Limit your time alone with that person. If the person is the one God has created to be your life-time partner, then the relationship will stand the test of time.

I must warn you, though, that you'll still find some rotten eggs in Christian fellowship!

Much to my sorrow, I know a lot of teenagers who go to church with their parents but their hearts aren't there. Then they get into the youth groups, or singles groups, and pass around their bad habits, from drugs to sex! Before you know it, there's a whole group that thinks they're "getting away" with something!

So you may have to look hard for friends who play it straight! Don't settle for less!

In this evil age we're living in, the happiest marriages are the ones with Jesus Christ at the center.

I've talked to a lot of young adults who are single and lonely. They can't seem to find the right person for marriage.

My advice is to go to Bible studies and attend church regularly! THAT is where you'll find the right kind of marriage partner; not in the local bars!

You must learn to trust God's timing. It's

ALWAYS right!

In the meantime, have a good time with your friends. It's the only time in your life that you don't have to worry about paying the bills, picking the kids up at school or running errands!

Don't spoil this very special time with lust!

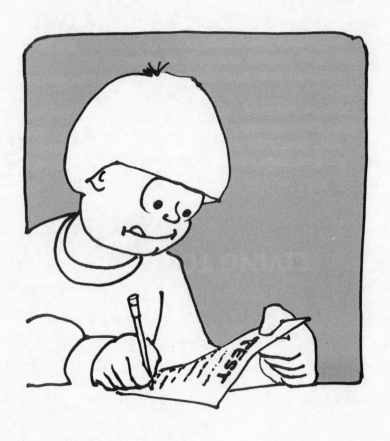

8

THE LOVE TEST

Recently the NBC Television Network did a special report on single women.[1] In this report, pre-marital sex was a major topic.

Several men were interviewed and they were all very honest. Their general attitude was that they had sex with anyone who wanted it. They plainly said that this *didn't* mean they were committed to, or in love with, the person. It was just something they both decided to do.

One of the girls talked about a relationship she had.

They had both said, "I love you" many times, and were sleeping together. She was sure they would get married someday. Gradually, she noticed that he began looking at other women more and more.

After they broke up she realized that her "I love you" was not the same as his "I love you."

Then NBC interviewed her ex-boyfriend. He said that his "I love you" meant that she was the most special person in his life; that he respected her and thought she was a great lover. He never planned to marry her!

When the standard marriage vows were written centuries ago they were written with commitment: "... for richer or poorer, in sickness and in health ... "

This is true love. It isn't based on looks or actions. It's based on caring for someone else more than yourself. You want the very best for that person.

Falling in love is much easier for girls.

Give a girl a nice guy who will give her attention and affection, and she can grow to be very attached to him.

It's not as easy for guys.

They aren't as interested in what the girl likes as they are in "how far they can go."

It's like the old "macho" image that wants to "conquer" a girl by getting her in bed!

A study conducted by the Stress and Cardiovascular Research Center of St. Petersburg, Florida, has revealed that girls don't know how to say "no" and boys feel pressured to get them to say "yes." They found that the highest stress factor in a teenager's life is sex![2]

Just the other day I was with two guys who are seniors. They are going to a fine college next fall. The one guy is seriously seeing a girl. It seems like all he thinks or talks about is her. She's very pretty and well built.

I thought, "Man, he seems pretty committed to Cheryl."

Then I heard him say to this other guy, "Yeah, I can't wait to go to college. There are some foxy chicks in that big city!"

"Shh ... Cheryl's right over there ... ," said the other guy.

I had to laugh to myself! Some commitment!

It made me wonder if girls can find *any* commitment from anyone, unless the guy's 100 percent sold out to Jesus! *Those* guys know how to love, because they know Him who is love.

I'll complete this chapter with a few simple questions for you.

Test your relationships with these:

1. *Is he or she pushy for sex?*

2. *Does he or she try to get you alone in a tempting place?*

3. *Does he or she avoid you when you have a problem?*

4. *Is he or she looking at other guys or girls?*

5. *Does he or she make fun of you or the way you are?*

6. *Is he or she rude to you and wants his or her own way?*

If you have true love, both of you will say *no* to all the above questions.

[1] *2nd Thoughts On Being Single: NBC,* April 25, 1984

[2] *Bob Larson Reports:* May/June 1984

9

LIVING TOGETHER

One popular view of many modern-day thinkers is that marriage has, of late, become an option. The "open minded" person should consider living together as an alternative to the traditional marriage.

Many have even suggested that it should be the first step before marriage is considered.

In Europe living together has become the popular alternative to marriage.

In Sweden it has become so common that two people living together is simply referred to as a "Stockholm marriage."

Even some religious groups say that living together is alright before marriage!

I suppose I have heard every argument possible to justify living together. "If we love each other, what difference does a piece of paper make?", is the age old argument.

In one of the most extensive polls ever taken, dealing strictly with teenagers, some 160,000 junior-and senior-high schoolers shared their views on living together.

The response was startling! Eighty percent of the boys, and almost seventy percent of the girls said they would live with someone before getting married![1]

It's easy to understand why the current generation is so afraid of getting married. A lot of them are from broken homes!

The current divorce rate averages about one out of every three ending in divorce.

But we should never think that because someone else has failed, we're going to fail at marriage, too! Anyone who wants a good marriage can have a good marriage; especially the Christian!

Is living together better than marriage?

Does living together prior to marriage give the relationship a better chance of making it?

Those who try it say that it will because they have the chance to adjust to their partner's living habits before tying the big knot!

Let's take a closer look at living together.

For 10 years, Dr. Nancy Moore Clatworthy, a 53-year-old sociologist at Ohio State University, has been studying the upturn in unmarried couples living together. She states that she began her research with a neutral opinion.

But her findings convinced her that it was not a good option to marriage.

When *Seventeen* magazine representatives,

Charles and Bonnie Remsberg , inquired of her study, she had the following to say about certain topics:[2]

RESPECT

"Among those who had married but lived together first, the most common problems were in the areas of adjustment, happiness, and respect. For instance, people were asked to check off the degree of respect.

"Those who had married first had a higher degree of respect than those who had lived together first."

HAPPINESS

"One question asked couples to estimate their usual level of personal happiness. One of the possible answers was 'extremely unhappy.' The only people who checked that answer were the ones who had lived together before marriage. None of the 'married firsts' checked that answer."

SEX

"We asked questions about finances, household matters, recreation, demonstration of affection, and friends. In every area, the couples who had lived together before marriage disagreed more often than the couples who had not. Invariably, the couples who had married first indicated a higher degree of unity on these day to day matters in their marriage."

But the finding that surprised Dr. Clatworthy most concerned sex.

Couples who had lived together before marriage disagreed more about sex than anything else.

"You'd assume that this would be an area that could be satisfactorily resolved in a living together period," she remarked. "But it usually isn't."

BREAKING UP

One of the questions was "How often do you fantasize breaking off with your spouse?"

One of the answers to this question was "often."

The only people who checked that answer had lived together before marriage! None of the people who had married first selected that answer.

Isn't it amazing that those who live together are supposed to be solving the problem of the tied-down feeling, yet they're the ones who fantasize most about breaking up?

CHEATING

After all, isn't one of the main reasons two people live together is so thay can satisfy each other sexually?

One would think so, but recent statistics from a survey of over 4,000 men show that men living with partners to whom they were not married seemed less committed to having sex only with their live-in partners. Approximately 66 percent (or two-thirds) admitted to cheating.

So it is clear that living together, in most cases, is simply easy sex and free companionship.

The serious thinker should consider these statistics before making any type of choice free from total commitment of marriage.

IS ANYTHING SOLVED BY LIVING TOGETHER?

"Almost half of the people who had lived together first said they had the same number of problems after marriage as before."

Dr. Clatworthy goes on to say, "Almost 20 percent said that after marriage they had more problems than before."

It is hard to imagine that everything good that is supposed to happen when you live together never happens in real life!

WHO GETS HURT?

Who gets hurt the most? Girls do!

In Dr. Clatworthy's study she discovered that the impact of a break-up among live-ins resulted in females bearing the most hurt.

"The girls felt more dominated, more bored, more infringed upon. They were more likely to feel that their personalities and their sex needs were incompatible to their partners. Many more girls than boys felt they had lost their identity in the relationship."

In all actuality, for the live-in there is little future for a lasting relationship.

Sociologists compiled statistics several years ago which indicate that 75 percent of those who live together break up.

To put it bluntly, living together is simply wanting the benefits of being married without having to pay the price.

The people who began to live together aren't convinced the relationship will last. After all, if it doesn't work they can just leave!

You can't "just leave" when you're married. A divorce will cost you anywhere from several hundred dollars to thousands! (And many celebrities will testify to that!)

Instead of committing by marriage to work the relationship out for a lifetime, we decide to treat each other like a retail item at the store. If the suit doesn't fit, after a few years, get rid of it!

It reminds me of a man I know who left his wife of 35 years.

He frankly says, "I gave her the first 35 years of my life, now I'm going to spend the next 35 doing what I want to do!"

How shallow! How grossly self-centered!

Certainly marriage is the most important commitment to another human we'll ever make in this life; but we don't have the right to "play house" with people's lives!

If the statistics don't convince you how bad living together is for people, I hope and pray you can care enough about that special person not to treat them as another "experiment" in your life!

I know someone will be reading this who is already living with a person, so I want to address that situation.

Beyond the statistics and basic caring for human life is the Word of God. As other chapters in this book explain, sex before marriage is a sin.

God *will not* bless a sexual relationship outside of marriage. You may feel your relationship is good and it may "seem" God is blessing it, but you're deceived. Hebrews 11:25 says "sin is pleasure for a season." And how well we should *all* know those Bible words "we will reap what we sow!"

For those of you living together, I give this advice:

1. The first thing you must do is put a stop to the sexual sin. If no sex means no relationship, then you're much better off without both!

2. If you believe you're headed toward getting married, decide to stop having sex until you do and repent of the sin. If there's true love there, you'll both be able to do that.

3. Some of you just feel trapped! Usually it is the girls. You got into this relationship in a weak moment and seem to be caught in it. You're miserable with the person and miserable without them. The only solution to this type is to put an end to the whole relationship. It will be painful at first but it's

the only way back to reality!

This relationship has become a physical and emotional crutch and is a lot like being an alcoholic. Every moment you stay in that situation is another moment of your life you've wasted!

The Bible says that "Jesus heals the broken-hearted," and He can and will heal that big hole in your heart from breaking up.

But don't hang around for Jesus to change your boyfriend or girlfriend. He wants to change you! Repentance means "to turn from sin and turn towards God." Repent today and let Jesus give you a new start.

4. I must also talk about those "platonic" live-ins. That is, the opposite sex who lives together for the convenience of it. You see this type of relationship on the television show "Three's Company."

None of the three are romantically involved but live together because it's cheaper. It's amazing how our society accepts this as a normal way of living!

But this is not right.

The Bible tells us to "abstain from all appearance of evil" (1 Thess. 5:22) and to "give no place to the devil" (Eph. 4:27).

But these live-ins are guilty of both. Anyone can tune in to this show and hear Jack making sexual remarks to his two female roommates! And this is not far from reality. How can that be helped when the girls walk around in skimpy p.j.'s and Jack shares their bathroom?

Single people are easily tempted with sex. Only the fool would place himself in a position that would double his temptations!

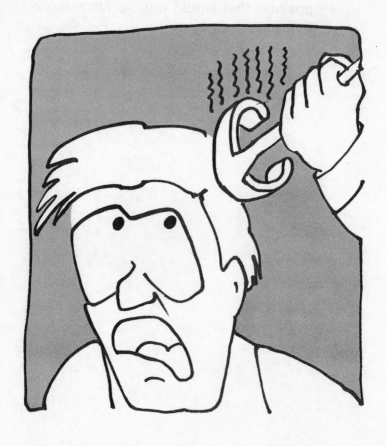

10

BRANDED

A college girl, who wrote to a very popular Christian magazine, said, "I was raised in a good Christian home.[1] I was always taught that sex before marriage was wrong. When my boyfriend and I began to get involved sexually, I felt guilty at first. Before long, I couldn't understand why I ever felt bad at all."

She went on to say that she and her boyfriend were not living together at college.

What was wrong with this confused college girl? She had ignored the warnings of her conscience until it finally gave up warning her!

The word conscience means "to know with." Broken down, CON means WITH, and SCIENCE means TO KNOW. So God has given us a conscience "to know with." Our consciences become sensitive alarms when they are set in time with the Word of God. Then, when we start to do something wrong, the alarm goes off, as if to say, "*Stop! This is wrong!*"

If we listen to our consciences, we become more sensitive to the Holy Spirit's voice as He seeks to control our minds. If we ignore our consciences, they get duller and harder to hear each time. Those who ignore it regularly, "sear" or "brand" it, as the scriptures say (1 Tim. 4:2).

It's like branding a cow. The ranchhands put a symbol on the cow with a hot iron. They say that you can take a long needle and stick it in the spot where the cow has been branded and the cow can't even feel it!

Well, this is what happened to that college girl. Her conscience was branded and she had no feelings of guilt. She no longer could tell the difference between right and wrong. So, she figures that means she's free! But she has been given a false peace.

Jesus talked about this kind of peace when He spoke of Satan in Luke 11:21, "When a strong man armed keeps his palace, his goods are in peace."

People, like this college girl, have given their palace, or body, to the strong man. In return he gives them a false peace.

Have you "seared" your conscience so you won't feel guilty? Have you given yourself over to this strong man?

Here are a few questions you can ask yourself to see if you have.

1. *Are you doing things now that you said you would never do?*

2. *Was there ever a time when you criticized others for doing what you are now doing?*

3. *Have you allowed a boy or girl to wear down your alarm on your conscience by going further and further sexually each time you are alone together?*

If the answer to any of the above questions is "yes," then you're on the road to destroying your conscience. You're so deep into sexual sin that you can't see how you could ever think as a virgin again!

I know one such girl. She had several lovers in her teenage years.

When Peggy came to know Christ in her late teens, she knew what she had been doing was evil. When she repented, God gave her conscience *new life*! At one point God brought this guy Mark into her life. They knew that God had put them together.

Peggy said that it wasn't too hard to keep from being physical, and she didn't have trouble forgetting her past.

She and Mark were both more hungry for God

than they were for each other!

But her problem was the future. She was afraid of having sex once they married because it had always been so dirty in her old life.

Peggy tells this beautiful story: "One night, just before my wedding day, I was crying before the Lord because I was scared about our wedding night. As I cried out, the Lord spoke to my heart so very clearly. He said that in *His* sight I *was* a virgin and that I would be like one to my husband. He told me that my marriage would be blessed by Him and that sex would be completely different than before I knew Jesus. I didn't understand how that could be, but I knew He had spoken to me. I had so much peace from that day on! I don't know how to explain it, but our wedding day was a true celebration and there was something so holy about our union. I was so surprised how we were like two virgins! We had so much fun, but yet the Spirit of God was there in our bedroom."

2 Corinthians 5:17 says: "Therefore, if any man be in Christ, he is a new creation: old things are passed away; behold, all things are become new."

11

— BRAINWASHED — BECOMING PURE AGAIN

Recently, while listening to the radio, I heard someone refer to a person who had become a Christian as being "brainwashed." The person responding said, "That's right! My brain needed some washing!"

Probably the most frustrating thing about being involved sexually before marriage is having to live with the memories. It seems to me that the greatest memorial that sin has is memories! Anytime Satan wants to discourage you or condemn you, he runs your past affairs through your mind as though you were at a movie!

I say this because I know what it is to do battle with thoughts about the past. Many of you who are now reading this book also know.

Someone once said it clearly: "Sex isn't in the

73

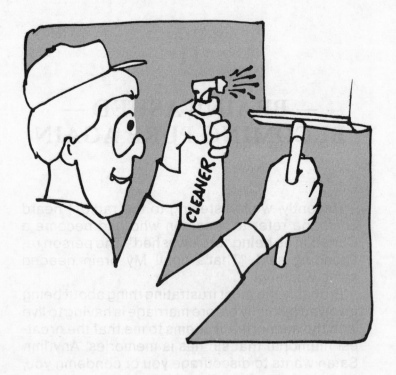

bed, it's in the head!"

The Apostle Paul said that the weapons we fight with are not physical but spiritual. And the battleground is the mind!

He goes on to say that we should cast down any imagination that exhalts itself against the knowledge that God has given us (2 Corinthians 10:4,5).

For the person who has been involved and now wants to become pure again, this is a battle he or she may have to fight many times. But I can testify that the victory can be won by the power of God through the direction of the Holy Spirit.

So, in this chapter, I would like to give you some steps in becoming free and pure in body and mind.

STEP I

Admit your sin to God. Tell Him exactly what you've done as if He didn't even know you had done it. This helps you to see and realize the seriousness of the sins you have committed.

Remember, all sin is a direct sin against God. This is no different.

STEP II

Repent.

Take steps that show you are turning from this sin and turning to God.

John the Baptist said, "Bring forth, therefore, fruits meet for repentance" (Matt. 3.8).

Show actions that are evidence of your repentance. For some of you these "fruits" may be cutting off some relationships or bad habits (sexual T.V. shows, movies, books). Show God, by your actions, how sorry you truly are.

STEP III

Renounce the sins of your fathers and forefathers.

This means to tell God that if there is any sin that has been in your family, or in your family's past generations, that you want it to stop with you.

The Bible tells us that it is possible for the sins of our forefathers to be passed on to us (Exodus 34:7).

This is especially true of immorality or sexual sins. Many times it has been in the family for many, many years.

STEP IV

Believe and receive the forgiveness of Christ. Thank Him for cleansing you by His suffering and by the shedding of His blood on the cross.

Realize that if He has forgiven you and accepted you, how can you do anything but forgive yourself? Sometimes we have a hard time believing He can forgive us. But He can and He does! Accept His forgiveness into your heart.

Don't forget the sinful woman He cleansed when He was alive was the same one He chose to appear to first after His ressurection! You are special to God!

STEP V

Don't let Satan condemn you! Most people don't know the difference between conviction and condemnation.

The Bible says, in Romans 8:1, "There is, therefore, now no condemnation to them who are in Christ Jesus, who walk not after the flesh, but after the Spirit."

This is the King James Version and some people argue that you must walk in the Spirit to be free from condemnation. But the original Greek it was written in, says, "There is, therefore, now no condemnation to those who are in Christ Jesus."

The only requirement is that you are a Christian. And if you are one, you can never be condemned; never!

I want to explain to you the difference between this conviction and condemnation. I will list their qualities.

CONDEMNATION

1. It is from Satan.

2. It is general and makes you feel bad about everything.

3. It makes you feel unworthy of receiving forgiveness from Christ. It discourages

you from coming before Him. Instead, it urges you to go back to your old ways because you can never be forgiven or live a Christian life. What a lie!

Do any of these things sound familiar? Notice that none of these give you hope or draw you back to Christ.

CONVICTION

1. It is done by the Holy Spirit.

2. It is specific. You don't feel bad about everything. He points out a specific area where you have sinned or fallen.

3. It draws you back to Christ. No matter what sin you commit, however terrible it may be, the Holy Spirit will always be drawing you back to Christ. Christ *always* wants to forgive you, cleanse you and fill you with His powerful love! The Holy Spirit will never make you feel discouraged or unworthy to receive forgiveness.

Now you must act on these truths. Tell Satan you will never allow him to condemn you again. *If* you should ever fall again, review this chapter and take a stand against that sin.

Do you know why Satan always uses the past on you? That's all he knows! God is the only one who knows your future. Because of this fact, Satan will always take your past and try to beat you over the head with it. If he can get you discouraged enough to go back to your old ways, then he can have some control over your future!

God forgets your past and gives you a bright future!

Learning the difference between conviction and condemnation is one of the most important lessons you will ever learn. It is the gateway to becoming pure again! Don't forget it!

> "But if we walk in the light, as he is in the light, we have fellowship one with another, and the blood of Jesus Christ cleanses us from all sin. If we confess our sins, he is faithful and just to forgive us our sins, and to cleanse us from all unrighteousness" (1 John 1:7,9).

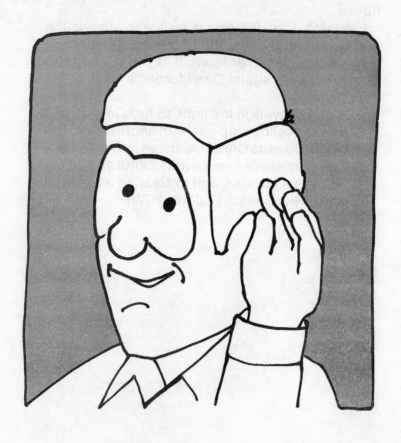

12

TRUE CONFESSIONS

The testimonies you are about to read are those of real people.

May God reward each of them for their honesty and for their desire to remember a painful past in order to help someone else from making the same mistakes!

SHARON

"When I was asked to write this, I was hesitant at first. But then I thought that if it might help convince one person not to sin, it would be worth it.

"During my years in high school, I was like my friends who were interested in doing whatever was fun and exciting. I knew there was a God, but I did my best not to think about Him!

"When I was about 15, I met this guy. He was

81

several years older than me, and much more mature than the high school guys. Anyway, we started dating and I thought he was so good looking. After a few dates he wanted to have sex, but I turned his offer down because I hardly knew him. As time went on, I began to get scared that he would find another girlfriend. And the fear of losing him was more than I could take; not because I loved him, but because I loved the attention and affection he gave me. Many of my friends were sleeping with their boyfriends, and a few were on the pill. So I started feeling like I was missing out on all the fun and excitment. Because of these two reasons, I decided to try it.

"Sex seemed fun, at first. But I never dreamed it would turn out so bad. Over the next year our relationship got worse and worse. He had a horrible temper, and I was always afraid of him. It was almost as if we hated each other! Several times I broke up with him, but we always ended up together again. All he had to do was put his arms around me and I would go back to him. The physical attachment was so strong! I guess it's like the Bible says, that when two people are joined together, they become one flesh.

"I took a lot of physical and emotional abuse from him. What was so strange is the fact that I never loved him! He had just been an experiment that made me miserable, yet I couldn't give it up.

"Finally, I was able to break up with him for good. Six months later I gave my life to the Lord and He forgave me for all this sin.

"Please, don't get involved in sex! Let the Lord

fill the empty spaces of your life. He will be your best friend if you let Him."

BILL

"I met my old girlfriend at church. We were going to church with our families. Both of us were very lonely and didn't feel like anyone cared about us. We were starved for love and affection. Since we were two of a kind, we hit it right off and started dating. We just hung out alone, because we didn't have a lot of friends. It was two years before we had sex. When we finally did, it just kinda happened; I guess because we were alone together all the time.

"We each knew it was wrong, but we didn't want to hurt each other's feelings. So it just went on and on. One thing that bothered me about it was that I didn't trust her. We talked on and off about getting married when she turned 18. But I thought if she wouldn't save herself until marriage for me what would keep her from cheating on me once we were married?

"I came to a point where I started getting serious about the Lord. I realized I'd never be happy without Jesus and that I needed to get straight. I told Tracy that our relationship had to change. So she started dating other guys! Within a year she ended up marrying some guy because she got pregnant. Then she has a miscarriage and was trying to get a divorce because she really didn't love him.

"Jesus has really changed me. I'm not worried about having a girlfriend now. I know that, when the time is right, He'll give me a wife to share my life with."

LESLIE

"I became a born-again Christian as a young teenager, but I was not serving the Lord when I became engaged. I always felt that I didn't want to have sex before marriage. I wanted to wait until I was married.

"We necked and petted knowing we were going to be married anyway. But then my sister asked me if we were having sex. She said that she did it before they were married. She made it seem exciting and off limits. The thought came into my head, 'if my sister did it, why can't I?' I convinced myself it was okay because we were getting married.

"When we finally went to bed, I felt tense, uncomfortable, and guilty. It was a let down and not at all how I expected it to be. Instead of tenderness, we were in a hurry. Instead of love, there was guilt. I cried and all I could think about was that I wasn't a virgin anymore. I wanted our wedding night to be so special. I felt dirty and, even though I was going along with it as much as he was, I felt used. I lost my respect for myself and for him. I felt that, just by looking at me, other people knew what had happened. There was a loss of innocence, not in a beautiful way, (as I know it would have been in God's plan), but in an ugly way.

"God is faithful to forgive but I still remember the pain, and regret what I did."

GREG

"I remained a virgin until I got out of high school

and began working as a chef at a restaurant. Word got around and, before I knew it, a race began between the waitresses to see who could break my virginity! Since they came after me, not wanting any commitment from me, I just thought of sex as a recreation, like sports. Once I had it, I became hooked and had a lot of affairs for the fun of it.

"There wasn't any emotional attachment except once. One girl wanted to marry me and I was really sorry but I didn't love her!

"Shortly after that I got saved. I realized that sex before marriage was a sin.

"Sometime later, God brought my wife into my life. She was a virgin. Because I had so much lust in my prior sexual experience, it was hard to adjust to having an inexperienced sex partner. Things would've been so different if I would've saved myself just for her! But, because I didn't wait, I had to discipline my flesh and put down old lustful feelings. God has healed me in this area, but it was a painful process. Take my advice and save yourself for God's chosen partner for your life!"

"And I find more bitter than death the woman whose heart is snares and nets, and her hands as bands; whoso pleases God shall escape from her; but the sinner shall be taken by her" (Ecclesiates 8:26).

LINDA

"I was 16 years old and he was my 'first love.' I say love here, but I really had a bad case of lust! I thought it was love. After all, everytime I heard his voice my heart jumped!

"He was my best friend's brother and a real Mr. Macho. When he wanted to go to bed, I thought it was expected of me. My best friend convinced me it was an act of two people who had something very special. She said parents, and others, who said 'don't do it', just didn't understand this special type of love. But I don't blame her. I made the choice and it was my mistake. Not too long after that, the Lord allowed me to see it was a selfish act and a sinful one that hurt Him. So I broke up with him. He cried and said he really loved me and wanted to marry me. But I knew already that he was too selfish to really love me. Then I failed to draw close to the Lord and repent like I should've. So, in search for love and acceptance, I fell into the same trap a couple more times!

"Finally, when I was so miserable and feeling very used, I came to the Lord and repented. He made me feel loved and accepted by Him. I was sad to realize I could've had his love and acceptance all along! Anyway, He forgave me of my sin and took away all the condemnation. He helped me to learn how to forgive and love myself. He gave new life to my burned-out conscience. I learned that true love chooses what is best spiritually, physically and mentally for the other person.

"I am now engaged to a wonderful Christian guy who really loves me. At first he really had a problem dealing with the fact that I was not a virgin. He saved himself for his wife and couldn't understand why I hadn't done the same. I had really fooled myself by thinking there was no one better to wait for! Satan had really blinded me!

"My fiancee was very hurt and I was sick that I had hurt this special person. All along God wanted me to obey Him so that I would be a precious and untouched gift to this guy who I now so deeply love!

"If you're reading this now and are going through a heavy relationship, remember that if you disobey God you set yourself on a road full of hurt, pain, and rejection. God only wants us to obey Him, so He can give us His best!"

CHARLENE

"My dad died when I was 12 and from that point on I was always trying to get guys to like me. When I first started dating in my early teens the different guys were always trying to get me to go all the way but I was scared. Eventually, by the age of 15, one guy came along who was very forceful. He insisted we go to bed and I couldn't resist him. From that time on I clung to him like a puppy dog. I was afraid no one else could ever care about me even though I knew *he* really didn't love me. I had some bad experiences with drugs and ended up running far away from home and him.

"In my new world I realized that I had become a woman and that I could use my sexuality to get whatever, or whoever, I wanted. I was really shocked to see this work! It was a real game to me.

"Then one day I woke up and realized that nothing had any value to me. I had everything anyone could ever ask for but it meant nothing to me. All my friends envied me but I was miserable.

"Eventually I came to know Jesus and my whole

world changed. I finally understood how sinful I'd been and how precious sex is in God's sight. I was so ashamed that I had used it like a toy. I didn't know how I could ever have sex again and feel good about it. But God worked a miracle and gave me a husband who loved Him. We have both had immoral pasts but God made us feel clean and new."

13

A PERSONAL MESSAGE TO GUYS

God has given you a special role in your relationship with girls. She will look to you for leadership and direction. If you take advantage of that position, God will hold you personally responsible.

In most situations your girlfriend will do exactly what you want her to do. This is because her natural desire is to please you and make you happy.

Many guys misinterpret that to mean that a girl wants to be sexually involved. This is not the case at all.

Girls are more concerned with wanting someone to like their personality than they are with wanting physical contact.

In almost all cases, when a couple gets involved physically, it's at the guy's insistence. Then, even when a girl does "give in" it's only because she wants his acceptance.

Girls are afraid that if they say "no" they'll make the guy feel the rejection they themselves so greatly fear. If you do take advantage of her, you will be showing her that you really cannot be trusted. In the end she *will* be rejecting you because you took advantage of her love.

Do you want to marry a virgin? What makes you think that she wants anything less? She wants to marry someone who has been waiting for her and not willing to jump in bed with anyone who seemed capable of adding some new thrill to life!

Just think about all the things you want your girlfriend, or future wife, to be like. Do you meet the high standards you are expecting from her? If you don't, either you need to change your expectations or your expectations need to change you.

Remember, if you're waiting for a princess, she is also waiting for a prince. Don't run around just looking for someone so you don't have to be alone. Wait, and let God bring that special person into your life in His timing.

I remember when I was looking for someone special that I might spend the rest of my life with. Everywhere I went, in the back of my mind I was thinking, "God, is she here?"

After a long period of frustration I gave up!

I said "God, I am tired of trying to do your work. You bring the person you have for me into my life in your own timing."

Just over a year later, God did bring someone into my life. She is far better than any dream or expectations I ever had!

Guys, trust God and He will do the same for you!

14

A PERSONAL MESSAGE TO GIRLS

God has given you a beautiful and wonderful gift. As Eve completed Adam so you, too, can complete a man. You are to guard yourself as a treasure; one to be presented as a wedding gift to your husband. No matter how much you feel you care for someone, sex is intended for marriage.

Don't let some guy cheat you! Most of them will tell you anything you would like to hear just to get what they want from you. Remember, a guy will give love to get sex. So be sure his love is genuine and intended for marriage before you say "I love you."

Don't let everyone around you make you think you're wierd if you don't have a boyfriend. It's more important to wait for the right guy than to ruin it for that right guy because you didn't want

I

your friends to think you were a jerk!

Friends can be replaced; your virginity cannot! Once you have given up your virginity to someone it can never be regained.

In all my travels across the world I have not met one guy yet who didn't want to marry a virgin. They may have wanted to spend the night with an experienced girl but they never wanted to spend their life with one!

Sometimes a guy will even threaten a girl by saying, "If you really love me, you'll have sex with me. If you don't love me, we may as well break up."

In almost every case, where the girl has given in, the guy eventually breaks up with her. If he really loved her, he would respect her for refusing to be "loose" with something so precious!

God has a plan for your life. In that plan he has a man just right for you. Save yourself for that person and God will bless you beyond your wildest dreams!

MORE FAITH-BUILDING BOOKS BY HUNTINGTON HOUSE

GLOBALISM: AMERICA'S DEMISE, By William Bowen, Jr., $8.95 (hard back). The Globalists — some of the most powerful people on earth — have plans to totally eliminate God, the family and the United States as we know it today.

Globalism is the vehicle the humanists are using to implement their secular humanistic philosophy to bring about their one-world government.

This book clearly alerts Christians to what the Globalists have planned for them.

MURDERED HEIRESS . . . LIVING WITNESS, by Dr. Petti Wagner, $5.95. This is the book of the year about Dr. Petti Wagner — heiress to a large fortune — who was kidnapped and murdered for her wealth, yet through a miracle of God lives today.

Dr. Wagner did indeed endure a horrible death experience, but through God's mercy, she had her life given back to her to serve Jesus and help suffering humanity.

Some of the events recorded in the book are terrifying. But the purpose is not to detail a violent murder conspiracy but to magnify the glorious intervention of God.

THE HIDDEN DANGERS OF THE RAINBOW: The New Age Movement and Our Coming Age of Barbarism, by Constance Cumbey, $5.95. A national best-seller, this book exposes the New Age Movement which is made up of tens of thousands of organizations throughout the world. The movement's goal is to set up a one-world order under the leadership of a false christ.

Mrs. Cumbey is a trial lawyer from Detroit, Mich., and has spent years exposing the New Age Movement and the false christ.

TRAINING FOR TRIUMPH: A Handbook for Mothers and Fathers, by Dr. W. George Selig and Deborah D. Cole, $5.95. Being a good mother and father is one of life's great challenges. However, most parents undertake that challenge with little or no preparation, according to Dr. Selig, a professor at CBN University. He says that often, after a child's early years are past, parents sigh: "Where did we go wrong?"

Dr. Selig, who has 20 years of experience in the field of education, carefully explains how to be good mothers and fathers and how to apply good principles and teachings while children are still young.

Feel Better and Live Longer Through: THE DIVINE CONNECTION, by Dr. Donald Whitaker $4.95. This is a Christian's guide to life extension. Dr. Whitaker of Longview, Texas, says you really can feel better and live longer by following Biblical principles set forth in the Word of God.

THE DIVINE CONNECTION shows you how to experience divine health, a happier life, relief from stress, a better appearance, a healthier outlook, a zest for living and a sound emotional life. And much, much more.

THE AGONY OF DECEPTION by Ron Rigsbee with Dorothy Bakker, $6.95. Ron Rigsbee was a man who through surgery became a woman and now through the grace of God is a man again. This book — written very tastefully — is the story of God's wonderful grace and His miraculous deliverance of a disoriented young man. It offers hope for millions of others trapped in the agony of deception.

THE DAY THEY PADLOCKED THE CHURCH, by E. Edward Roe, $3.50. The warm yet heartbreaking story of Pastor Everett Sileven, a Nebraska Baptist pastor, who was jailed and his church padlocked because he refused to bow to Caesar. It is also the story of 1,000 Christians who stood with Pastor Sileven, in defying Nebraska tyranny in America's crisis of freedom.

BACKWARD MASKING UNMASKED Backward Satanic Messages of Rock and Roll Exposed, by Jacob Aranza, $4.95.

Are rock and roll stars using the technique of backward masking to implant their own religious and moral values into the minds of young people? Are these messages satanic, drug-related and filled with sexual immorality? Jacob Aranza answers these and other questions.

SCOPES II/THE GREAT DEBATE, by Louisiana State Senator Bill Keith, 193 pages, $4.95.

Senator Keith's book strikes a mortal blow at evolution which is the cornerstone of the religion of secular humanism. He explains what parents and others can do to assure that creation science receives equal time in the school classrooms, where Christian children's faith is being destroyed.

WHY J. R. ? A Psychiatrist Discusses the Villain of Dallas, by Dr. Lew Ryder, 152 pages, $4.95.

An eminent psychiatrist explains how the anti-Christian religion of Secular Humanism has taken over television programming and what Christians can do to fight back.

YES, send me the following books:

_____ copy (copies) of **A Reasonable Reason To Wait** @ $3.50 =

_____ copy (copies) of **Globalism: America's Demise** @ $8.95 =

_____ copy (copies) of **Murdered Heiress . . . Living Witness** @ $5.95 =

_____ copy (copies) of **The Hidden Dangers of the Rainbow** @ $5.95 =

_____ copy (copies) of **The Divine Connection** @ $4.95 =

_____ copy (copies) of **The Agony of Deception** @ $6.95 =

_____ copy (copies) of **Training for Triumph** @ $4.95 =

_____ copy (copies) of **The Day They Padlocked The Church** @ $3.50 =

_____ copy (copies) of **Backward Masking Unmasked** @ $4.95 =

_____ copy (copies) of **Scopes II/The Great Debate** @ $4.95 =

_____ copy (copies) of **Why J.R.?** @ $4.95 =

Enclosed is: $ _____ including postage (please include $1 per book for

postage) for _____ books.

Name _____

Address _____

City and State _____ Zip _____

Mail to Huntington House, Inc., P.O. Box 53788, Lafayette, La. 70505

Telephone Orders: (318) 222-1350

RECOMMENDED READING

If you are single:

DOORWAYS TO DISCIPLESHIP
Winkie Pratney

A HANDBOOK FOR FOLLOWERS OF JESUS
Winkie Pratney

If you are married:

INTENDED FOR PLEASURE
Dr. Ed Wheat

LOVE LIFE
Dr. Ed Wheat

Also available by Jacob Aranza

A 60 min. cassette
"SEX BEFORE MARRIAGE"
LOVE OR LUST

This tape is a must for every single person.

To order send $5.95 to:
Aranza Outreach
429 Bellevue St.
Lafayette, La. 70506

ABOUT THE CO–AUTHOR

THERESA LAMSON

Theresa Lamson, and her husband Gary, have been teaching Bible studies since 1976. With a continuing theme on the moving of the Holy Spirit, they frequently teach seminars in the Dallas, Texas area. Based in Lafayette, Louisiana, with their three sons, they have been continually teaching, counseling, and ministering deliverance to the oppressed; particularly to those who have been involved in immorality.

They currently attend and are members of Bethel Assembly of God in Lafayette where they serve as counselors and instructors.

Jacob Aranza and Theresa Lamson welcome your response. If you would like to contact them, send your letters to:

Jacob Aranza
429 Bellevue
Lafayette, LA 70506

Theresa Lamson
P.O. Box 52109
Lafayette, LA 70505